Makeup Artist
my notebook of
MAKEUP

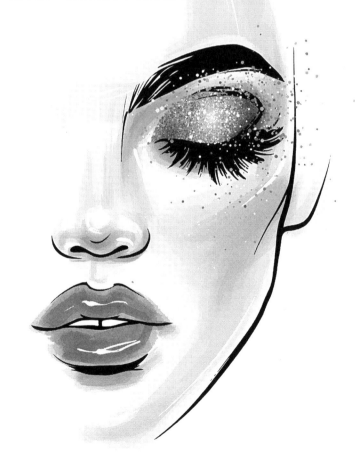

Tutorial of a PERFECT MAKEUP

Perfect makeup in 16 steps

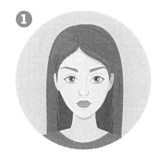

1. Clean your face

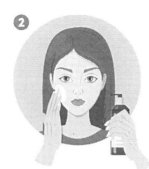

2. Apply sunscreen

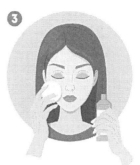

3. Wet the face

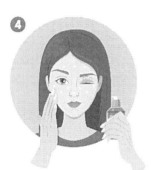

4. Add a primer

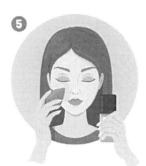

5. Apply the base

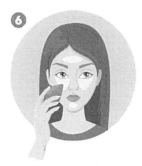

6. Adding a concealer

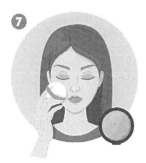

7. Apply the powder

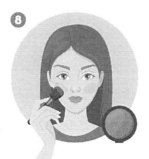

8. Apply the blush

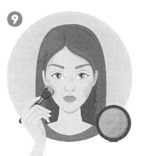

9. Apply a suntan cream

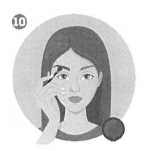
Fill in the browsers

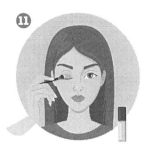
Apply a layer of eye candy

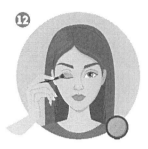
Apply an eye shadow

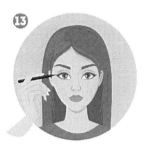
Apply eyeliner

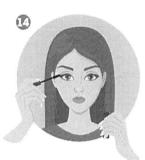
Apply mascara

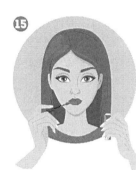
Apply a gloss

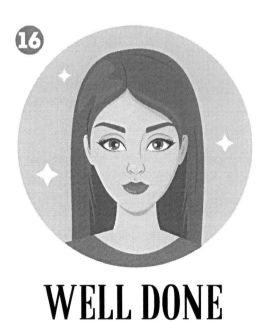

WELL DONE

Tips for the eyes

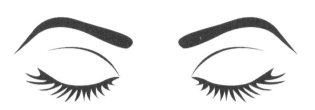

- Transform your classic eye pencil into an easy-to-apply gel pencil.

A classic green, black or burgundy khol pencil often draws a thin line that is difficult to apply. Place it under a flame for one second and let it cool for 15 seconds.

Your pencil now has the consistency of a gel pencil, allowing for a much smoother application.

- Perfect eyes !

Place the handle of the spoon along the outside corner of your eye to trace the tip of your doe's eye. Then, turn the spoon so that your eyelid is contained in the hollow of the spoon. Follow the outer contour of the spoon to create a clean circle and complete the outline of the doe's eye.

Fill in the drawn part, and there you are with professional eyes !

- It facilitates the use of the eyelash curler.

Gently heat your eyelash curler under your blow dryer until it is slightly warm (about 40/45°). The curl and hold of your lashes will last longer.

Juliette Bonne Aventure
Tous droits réservés

My makeup

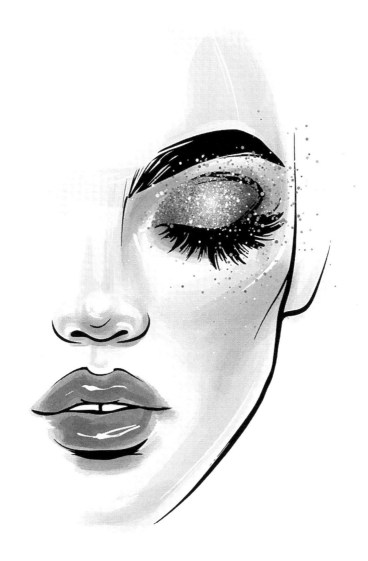

Skin preparation

Cleaning : ....
Scrubbing: ....
Lotion: ....
Moisturizing: ....
Base : ....
Foundation: ....
Correction: ....
Blush: ....
Powder: ....

Comments and advice

The eyes

Eyebrows: ....
Eyelids: ....
Pencil: ....
Mascara: ....
Liner : ....

The lips

Hydration: ....
balm ....
Gloss: ....
Pencil: ....

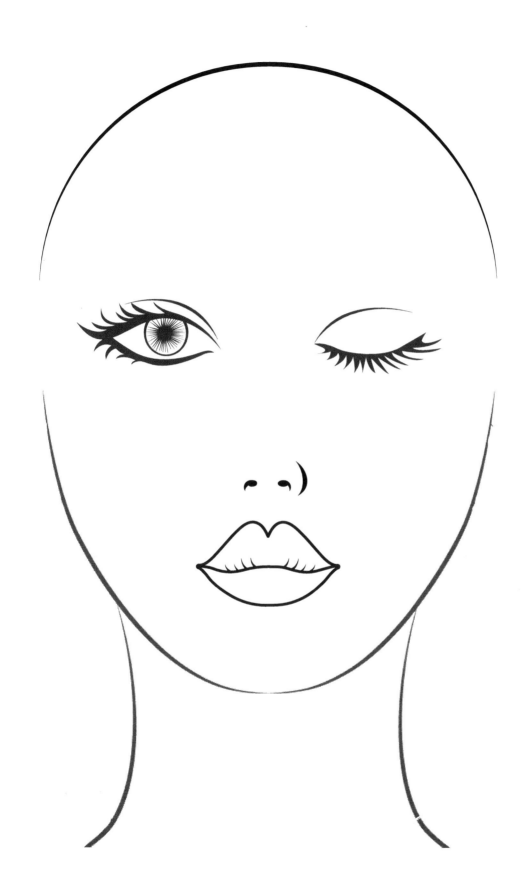

Skin preparation

Cleaning : _____
Scrubbing: _____
Lotion: _____
Moisturizing: _____
Base : _____
Foundation: _____
Correction: _____
Blush: _____
Powder: _____

Comments and advice

The eyes

Eyebrows: _____
Eyelids: _____
Pencil: _____
Mascara: _____
Liner : _____

The lips

Hydration: _____
balm _____
Gloss: _____
Pencil: _____

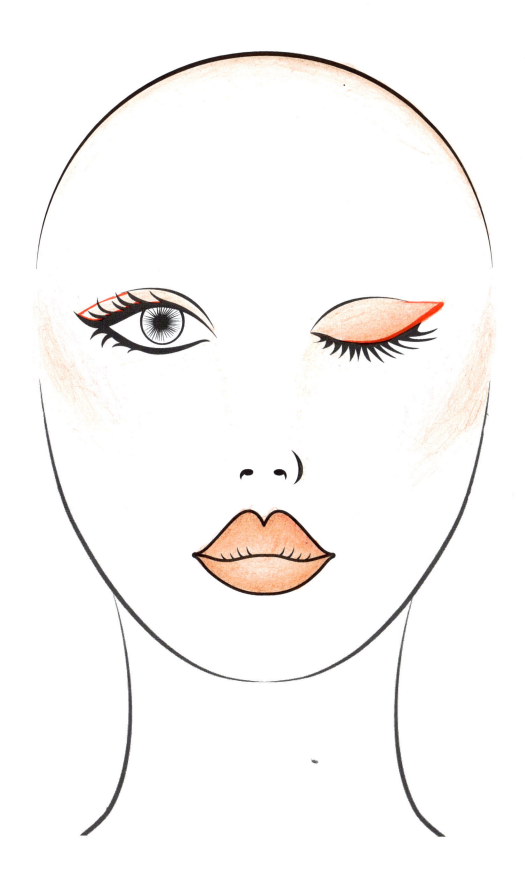

Skin preparation

Cleaning:
Scrubbing:
Lotion:
Moisturizing:
Base:
Foundation:
Correction:
Blush:
Powder:

Comments and advice

The eyes

Eyebrows:
Eyelids:
Pencil:
Mascara:
Liner:

The lips

Hydration:
balm
Gloss:
Pencil:

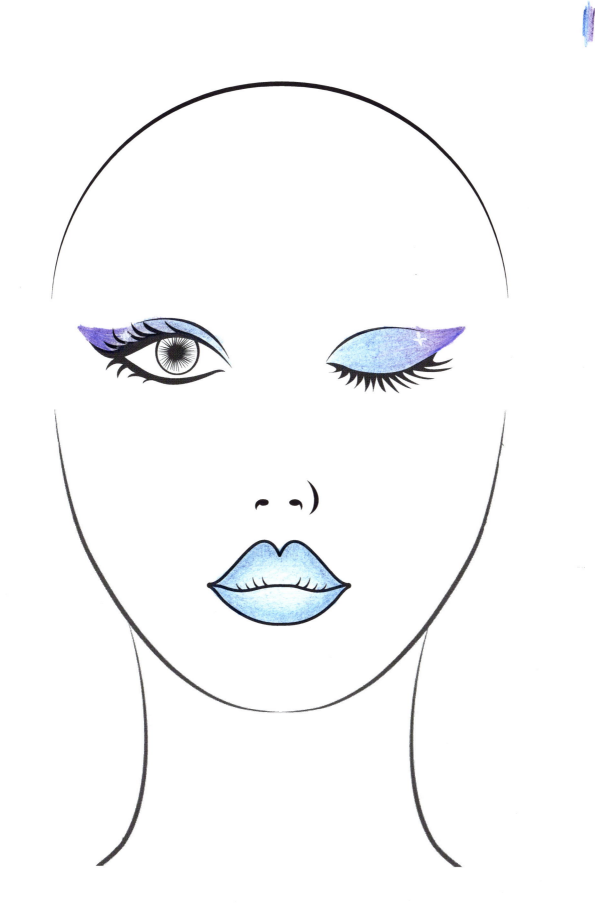

Skin preparation

Cleaning : ....
Scrubbing: ....
Lotion: ....
Moisturizing: ....
Base : ....
Foundation: ....
Correction: ....
Blush: ....
Powder: ....

Comments and advice

The eyes

Eyebrows: ....
Eyelids: ....
Pencil: ....
Mascara: ....
Liner : ....

The lips

Hydration: ....
balm ....
Gloss: ....
Pencil: ....

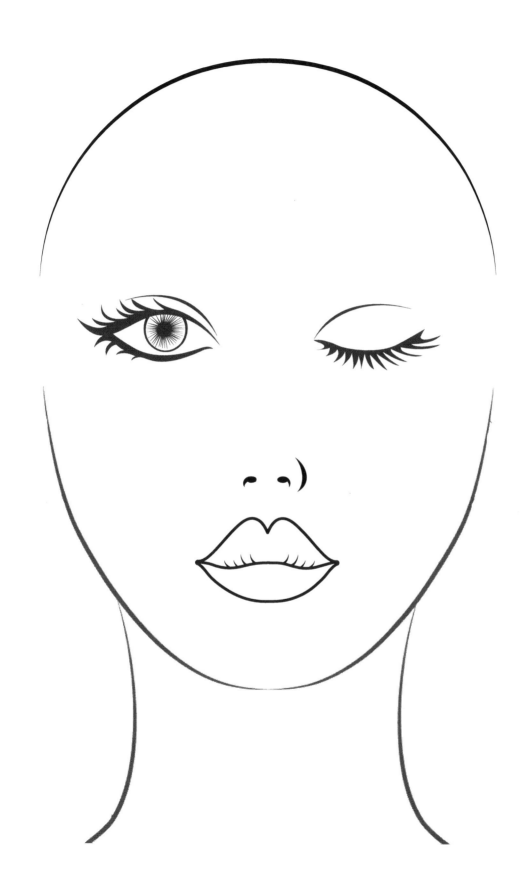

Skin preparation

Cleaning: _____
Scrubbing: _____
Lotion: _____
Moisturizing: _____
Base: _____
Foundation: _____
Correction: _____
Blush: _____
Powder: _____

Comments and advice

The eyes

Eyebrows: _____
Eyelids: _____
Pencil: _____
Mascara: _____
Liner: _____

The lips

Hydration: _____
balm _____
Gloss: _____
Pencil: _____

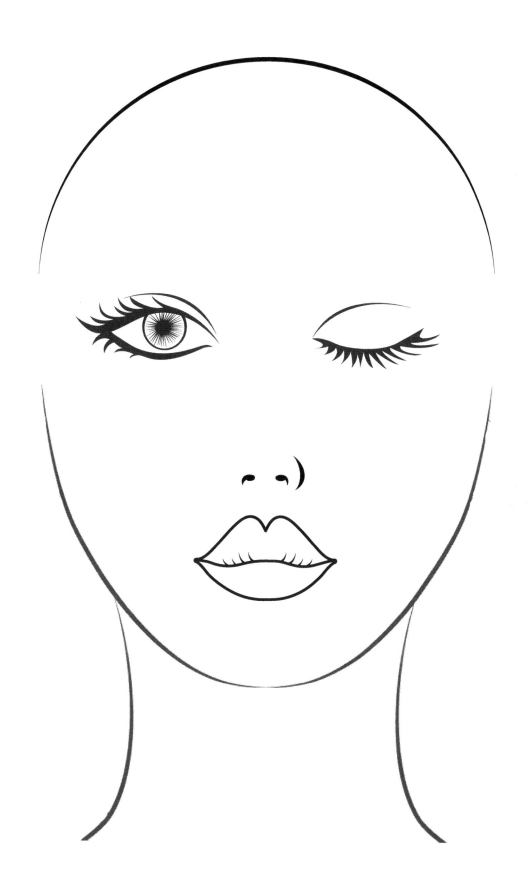

Skin preparation

Cleaning:
Scrubbing:
Lotion:
Moisturizing:
Base:
Foundation:
Correction:
Blush:
Powder:

Comments and advice

The eyes

Eyebrows:
Eyelids:
Pencil:
Mascara:
Liner:

The lips

Hydration:
balm
Gloss:
Pencil:

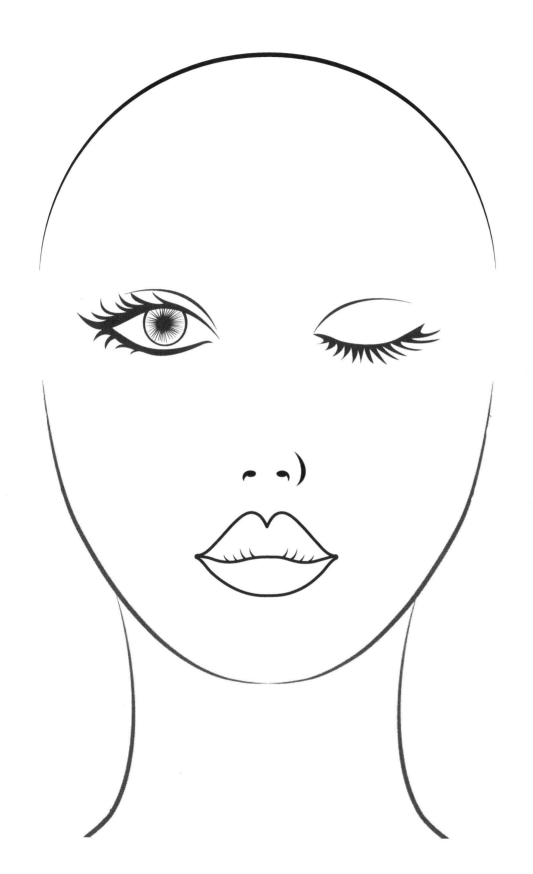

Skin preparation

Cleaning : _____
Scrubbing: _____
Lotion: _____
Moisturizing: _____
Base : _____
Foundation: _____
Correction: _____
Blush: _____
Powder: _____

Comments and advice

The eyes

Eyebrows: _____
Eyelids: _____
Pencil: _____
Mascara: _____
Liner : _____

The lips

Hydration: _____
balm _____
Gloss: _____
Pencil: _____

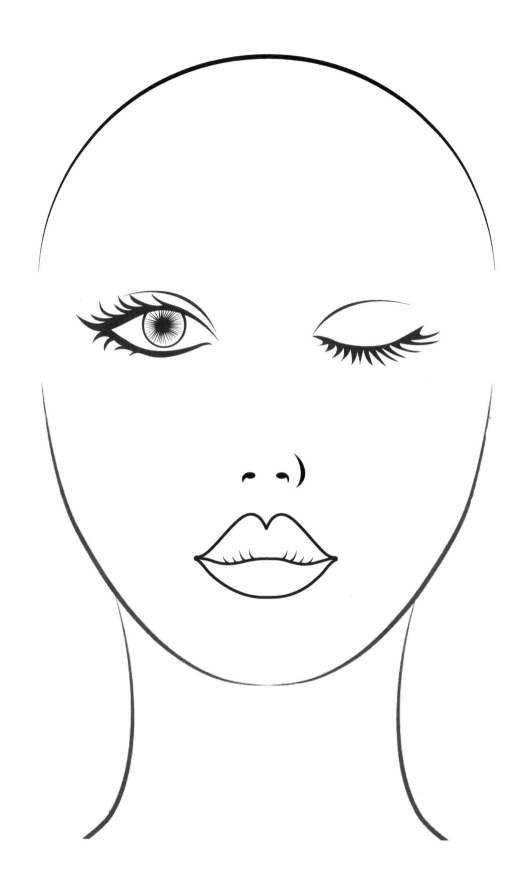

Skin preparation

Cleaning: ....

Scrubbing: ....

Lotion: ....

Moisturizing: ....

Base: ....

Foundation: ....

Correction: ....

Blush: ....

Powder: ....

Comments and advice

The eyes

Eyebrows: ....

Eyelids: ....

Pencil: ....

Mascara: ....

Liner: ....

The lips

Hydration: ....

balm ....

Gloss: ....

Pencil: ....

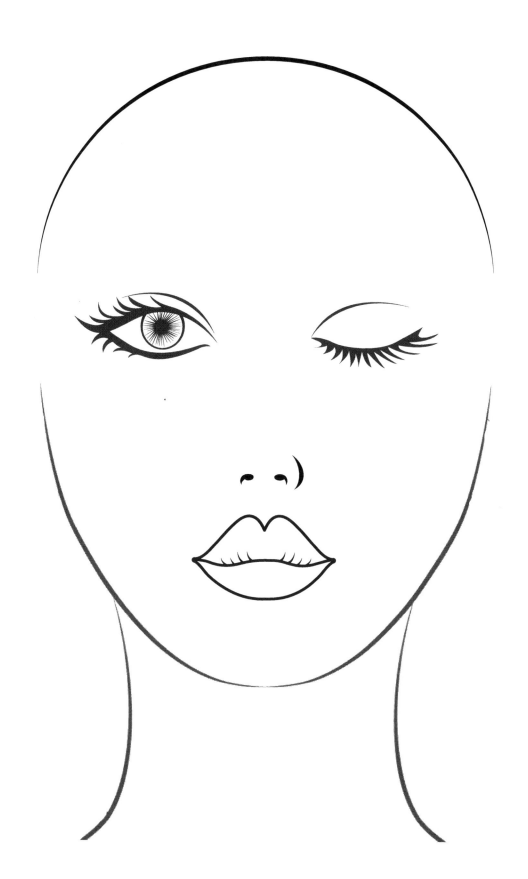

Skin preparation

Cleaning : _____

Scrubbing: _____

Lotion: _____

Moisturizing: _____

Base : _____

Foundation: _____

Correction: _____

Blush: _____

Powder: _____

Comments and advice

The eyes

Eyebrows: _____

Eyelids: _____

Pencil: _____

Mascara: _____

Liner : _____

The lips

Hydration: _____

balm _____

Gloss: _____

Pencil: _____

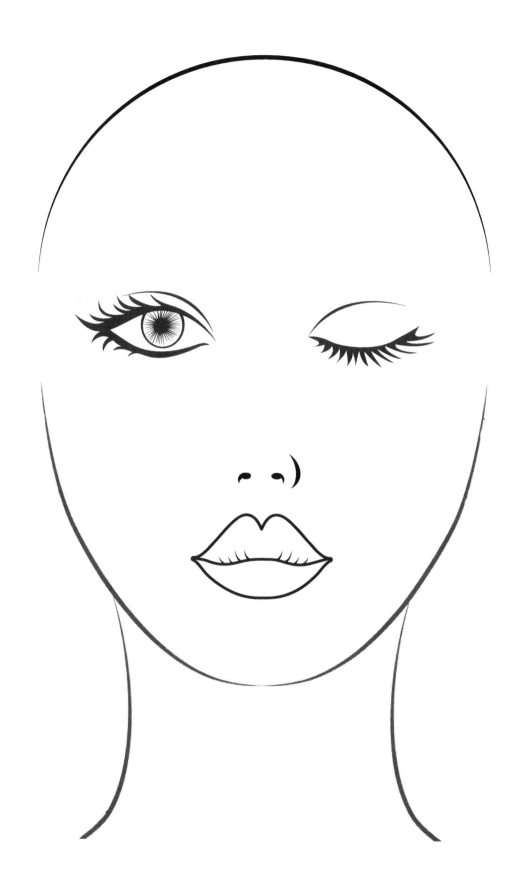

Skin preparation

Cleaning : _____
Scrubbing: _____
Lotion: _____
Moisturizing: _____
Base : _____
Foundation: _____
Correction: _____
Blush: _____
Powder: _____

Comments and advice

The eyes

Eyebrows: _____
Eyelids: _____
Pencil: _____
Mascara: _____
Liner : _____

The lips

Hydration: _____
balm _____
Gloss: _____
Pencil: _____

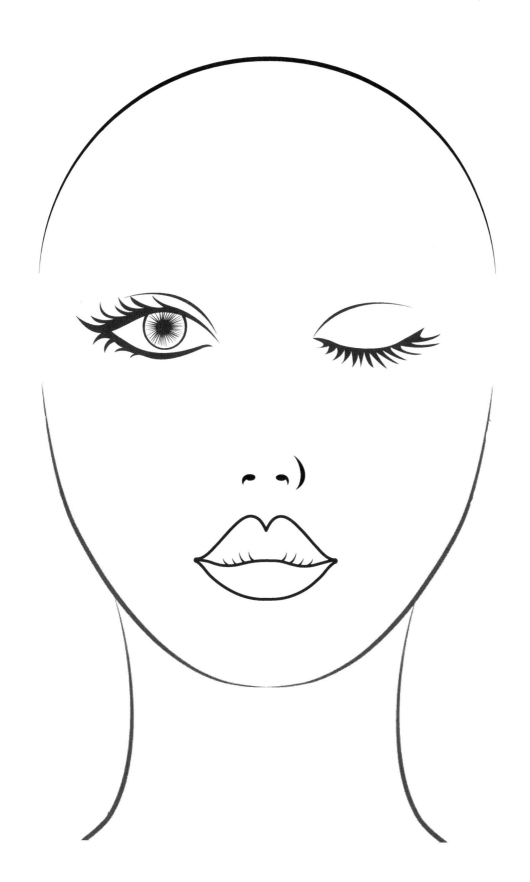

Skin preparation

Cleaning: _____
Scrubbing: _____
Lotion: _____
Moisturizing: _____
Base: _____
Foundation: _____
Correction: _____
Blush: _____
Powder: _____

Comments and advice

The eyes

Eyebrows: _____
Eyelids: _____
Pencil: _____
Mascara: _____
Liner: _____

The lips

Hydration: _____
balm _____
Gloss: _____
Pencil: _____

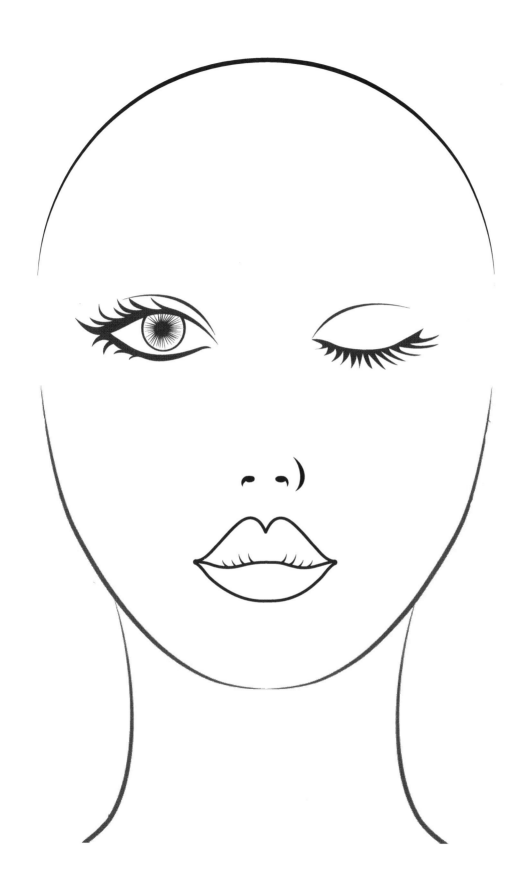

Skin preparation

Cleaning: ___
Scrubbing: ___
Lotion: ___
Moisturizing: ___
Base: ___
Foundation: ___
Correction: ___
Blush: ___
Powder: ___

Comments and advice

The eyes

Eyebrows: ___
Eyelids: ___
Pencil: ___
Mascara: ___
Liner: ___

The lips

Hydration: ___
balm ___
Gloss: ___
Pencil: ___

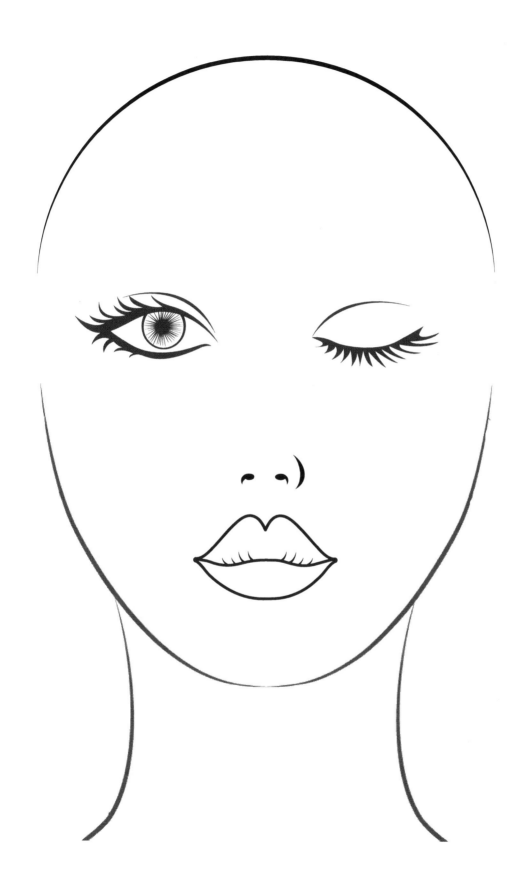

Skin preparation

Cleaning : ....

Scrubbing: ....

Lotion: ....

Moisturizing: ....

Base : ....

Foundation: ....

Correction: ....

Blush: ....

Powder: ....

Comments and advice

The eyes

Eyebrows: ....

Eyelids: ....

Pencil: ....

Mascara: ....

Liner : ....

The lips

Hydration: ....

balm ....

Gloss: ....

Pencil: ....

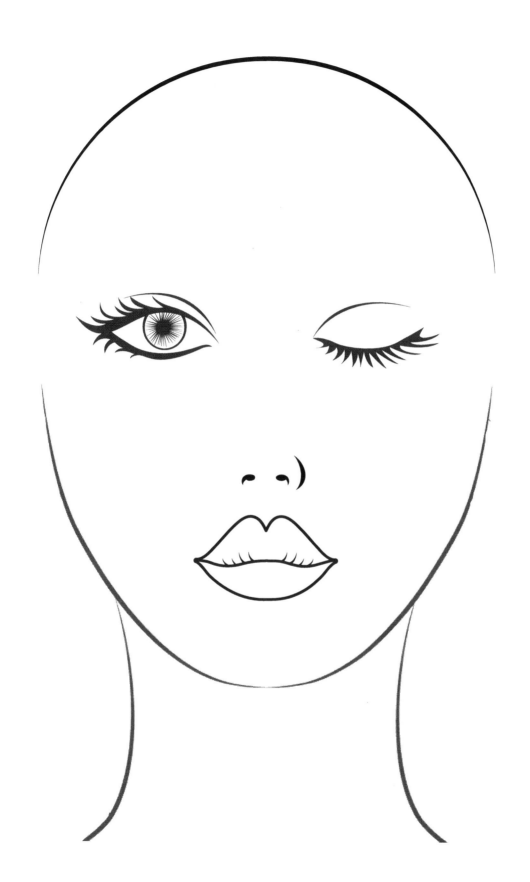

Skin preparation

Cleaning : _____

Scrubbing: _____

Lotion: _____

Moisturizing: _____

Base : _____

Foundation: _____

Correction: _____

Blush: _____

Powder: _____

Comments and advice

The eyes

Eyebrows: _____

Eyelids: _____

Pencil: _____

Mascara: _____

Liner : _____

The lips

Hydration: _____

balm _____

Gloss: _____

Pencil: _____

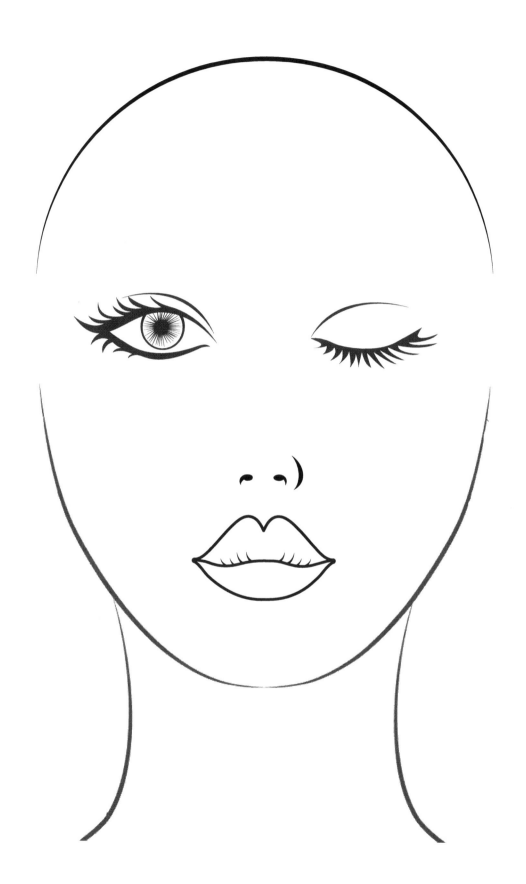

Skin preparation

Cleaning : ....

Scrubbing: ....

Lotion: ....

Moisturizing: ....

Base : ....

Foundation: ....

Correction: ....

Blush: ....

Powder: ....

Comments and advice

The eyes

Eyebrows: ....

Eyelids: ....

Pencil: ....

Mascara: ....

Liner : ....

The lips

Hydration: ....

balm ....

Gloss: ....

Pencil: ....

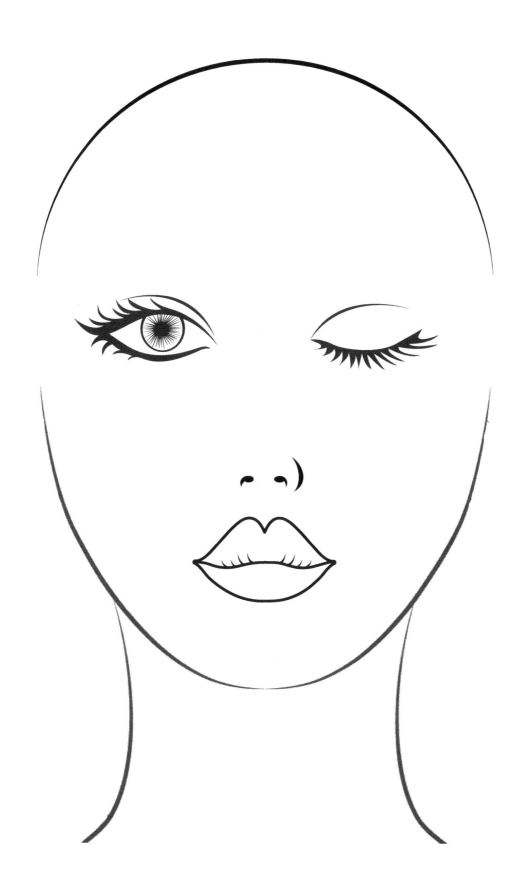

Skin preparation

Cleaning : ....
Scrubbing: ....
Lotion: ....
Moisturizing: ....
Base : ....
Foundation: ....
Correction: ....
Blush: ....
Powder: ....

Comments and advice

The eyes

Eyebrows: ....
Eyelids: ....
Pencil: ....
Mascara: ....
Liner : ....

The lips

Hydration: ....
balm ....
Gloss: ....
Pencil: ....

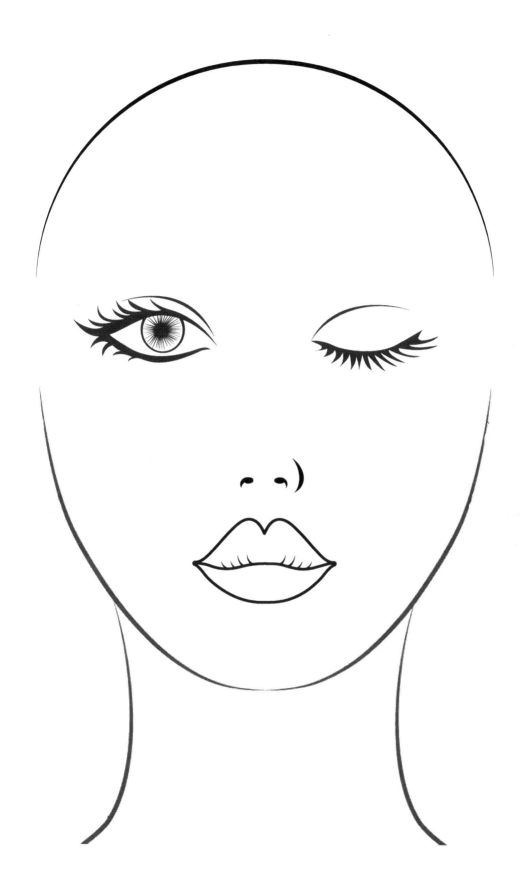

Skin preparation

Cleaning : _____

Scrubbing: _____

Lotion: _____

Moisturizing: _____

Base : _____

Foundation: _____

Correction: _____

Blush: _____

Powder: _____

Comments and advice

The eyes

Eyebrows: _____

Eyelids: _____

Pencil: _____

Mascara: _____

Liner : _____

The lips

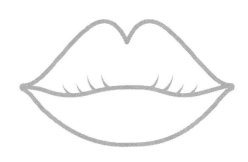

Hydration: _____

balm _____

Gloss: _____

Pencil: _____

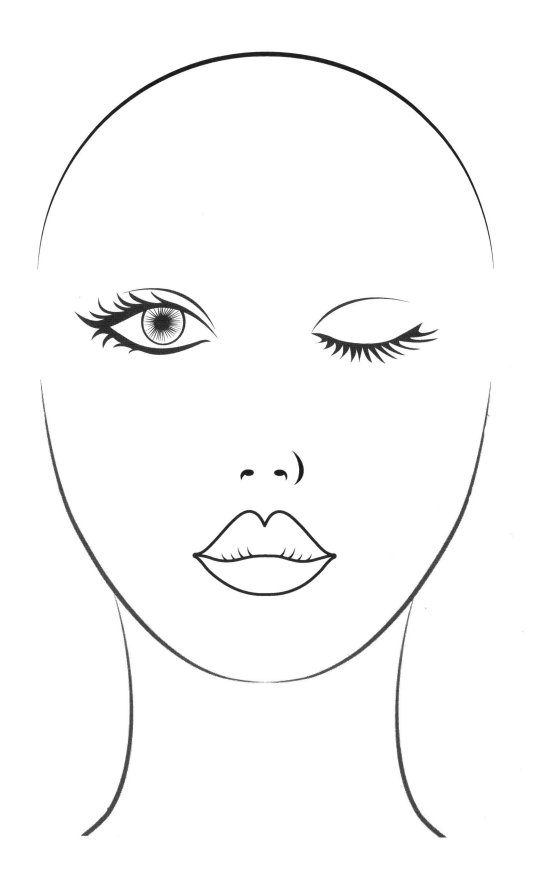

Skin preparation

Cleaning : _____
Scrubbing: _____
Lotion: _____
Moisturizing: _____
Base : _____
Foundation: _____
Correction: _____
Blush: _____
Powder: _____

Comments and advice

The eyes

Eyebrows: _____
Eyelids: _____
Pencil: _____
Mascara: _____
Liner : _____

The lips

Hydration: _____
balm _____
Gloss: _____
Pencil: _____

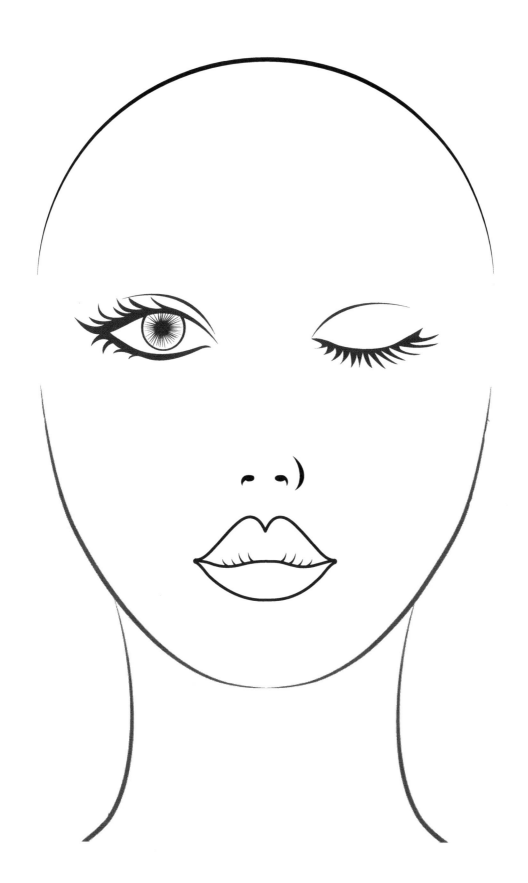

Skin preparation

Cleaning : _____

Scrubbing: _____

Lotion: _____

Moisturizing: _____

Base : _____

Foundation: _____

Correction: _____

Blush: _____

Powder: _____

Comments and advice

The eyes

Eyebrows: _____

Eyelids: _____

Pencil: _____

Mascara: _____

Liner : _____

The lips

Hydration: _____

balm _____

Gloss: _____

Pencil: _____

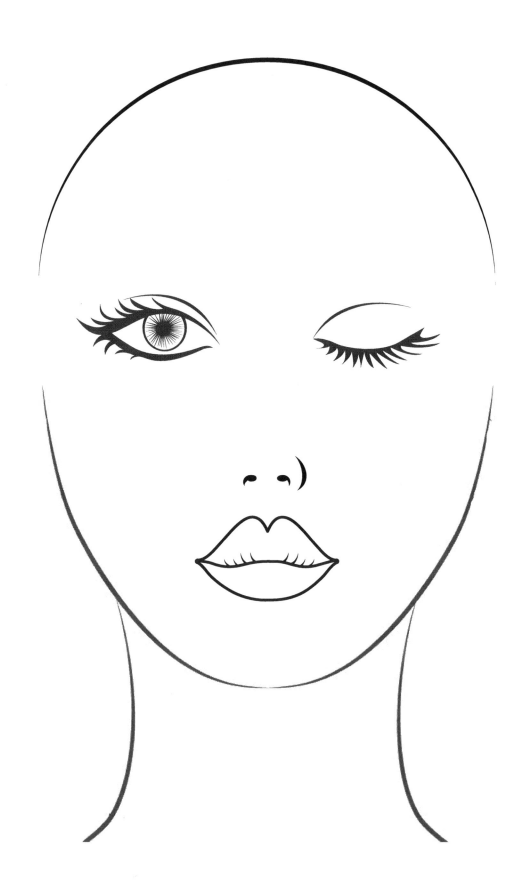

Skin preparation

Comments and advice

Cleaning : ....

Scrubbing: ....

Lotion: ....

Moisturizing: ....

Base : ....

Foundation: ....

Correction: ....

Blush: ....

Powder: ....

The eyes

Eyebrows: ....

Eyelids: ....

Pencil: ....

Mascara: ....

Liner : ....

The lips

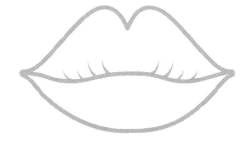

Hydration: ....

balm ....

Gloss: ....

Pencil: ....

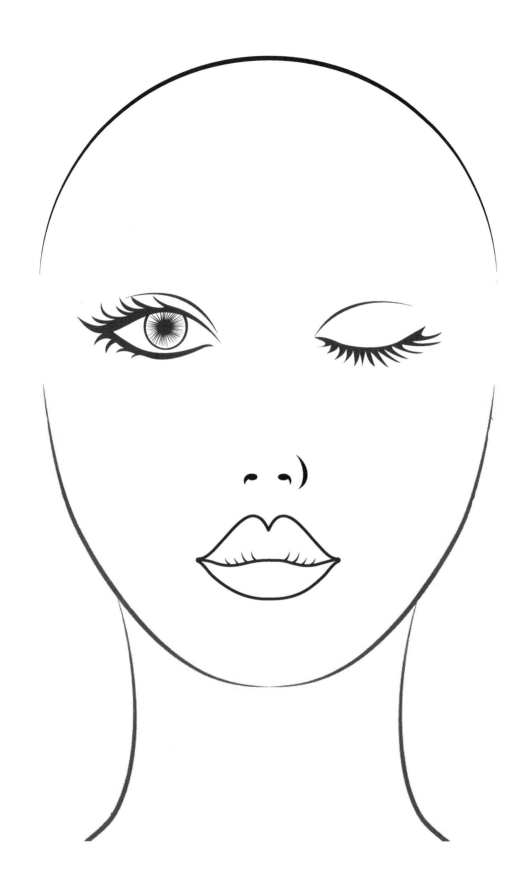

Skin preparation

Cleaning : ....
Scrubbing: ....
Lotion: ....
Moisturizing: ....
Base : ....
Foundation: ....
Correction: ....
Blush: ....
Powder: ....

Comments and advice

The eyes

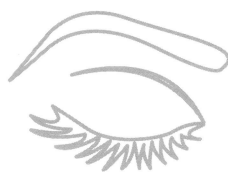

Eyebrows: ....
Eyelids: ....
Pencil: ....
Mascara: ....
Liner : ....

The lips

Hydration: ....
balm ....
Gloss: ....
Pencil: ....

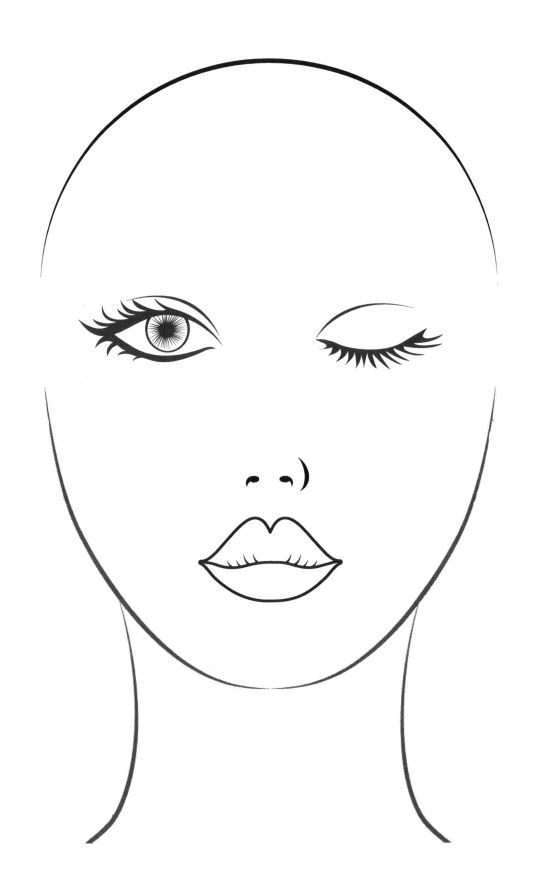

Skin preparation

Cleaning : _____
Scrubbing: _____
Lotion: _____
Moisturizing: _____
Base : _____
Foundation: _____
Correction: _____
Blush: _____
Powder: _____

Comments and advice

The eyes

Eyebrows: _____
Eyelids: _____
Pencil: _____
Mascara: _____
Liner : _____

The lips

Hydration: _____
balm _____
Gloss: _____
Pencil: _____

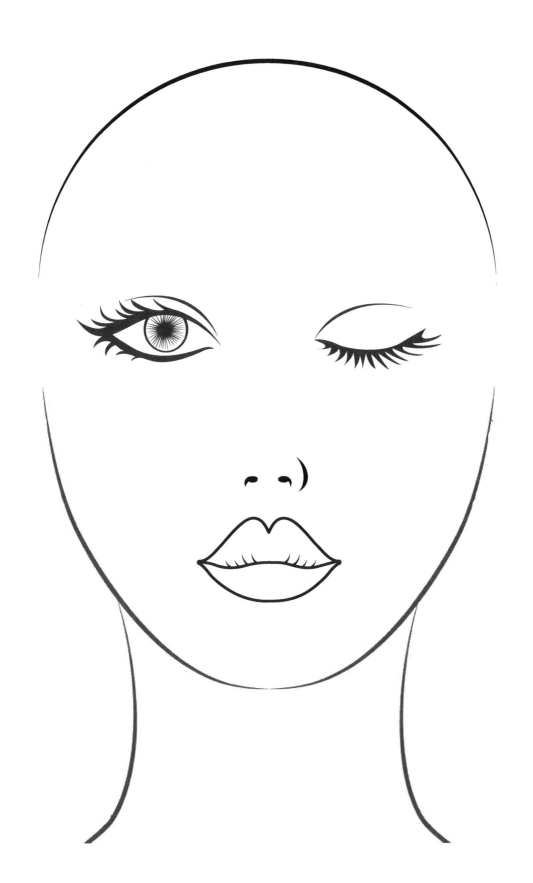

Skin preparation

Cleaning: ....
Scrubbing: ....
Lotion: ....
Moisturizing: ....
Base: ....
Foundation: ....
Correction: ....
Blush: ....
Powder: ....

Comments and advice

The eyes

Eyebrows: ....
Eyelids: ....
Pencil: ....
Mascara: ....
Liner: ....

The lips

Hydration: ....
balm ....
Gloss: ....
Pencil: ....

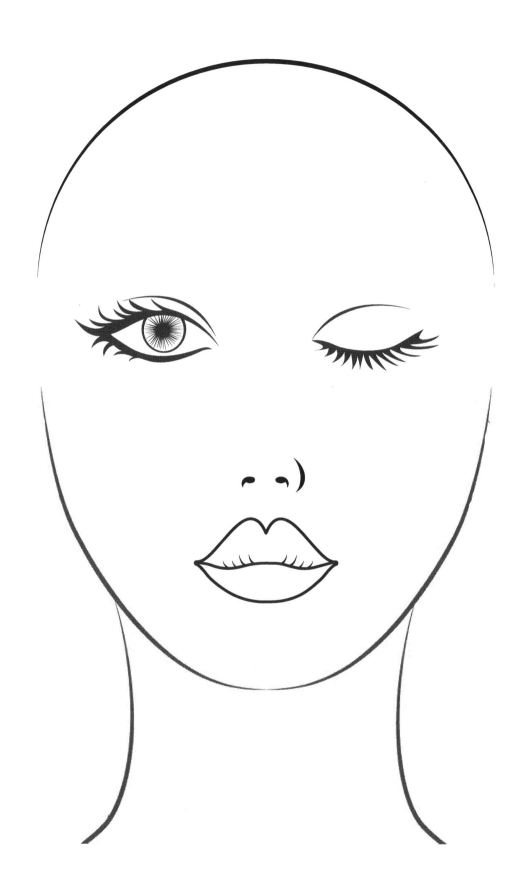

Skin preparation

Cleaning : _____

Scrubbing: _____

Lotion: _____

Moisturizing: _____

Base : _____

Foundation: _____

Correction: _____

Blush: _____

Powder: _____

Comments and advice

The eyes

Eyebrows: _____

Eyelids: _____

Pencil: _____

Mascara: _____

Liner : _____

The lips

Hydration: _____

balm _____

Gloss: _____

Pencil: _____

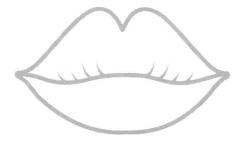

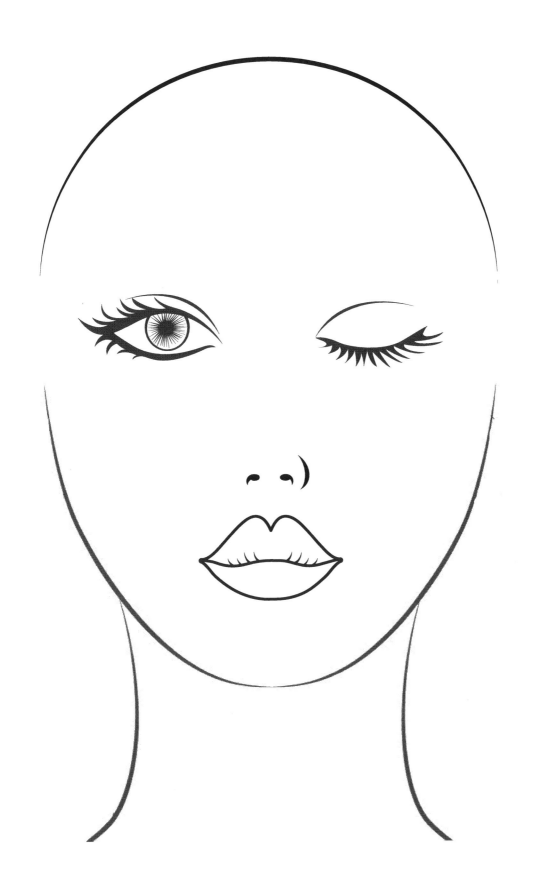

Skin preparation

Cleaning : ....

Scrubbing: ....

Lotion: ....

Moisturizing: ....

Base : ....

Foundation: ....

Correction: ....

Blush: ....

Powder: ....

Comments and advice

The eyes

Eyebrows: ....

Eyelids: ....

Pencil: ....

Mascara: ....

Liner : ....

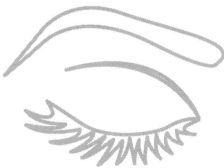

The lips

Hydration: ....

balm ....

Gloss: ....

Pencil: ....

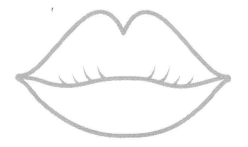

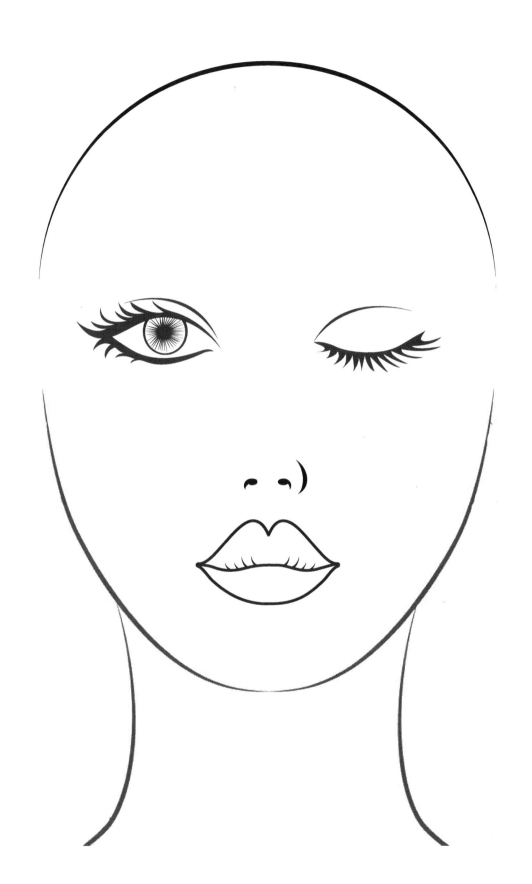

Skin preparation

Cleaning: ....

Scrubbing: ....

Lotion: ....

Moisturizing: ....

Base: ....

Foundation: ....

Correction: ....

Blush: ....

Powder: ....

Comments and advice

The eyes

Eyebrows: ....

Eyelids: ....

Pencil: ....

Mascara: ....

Liner: ....

The lips

Hydration: ....

balm ....

Gloss: ....

Pencil: ....

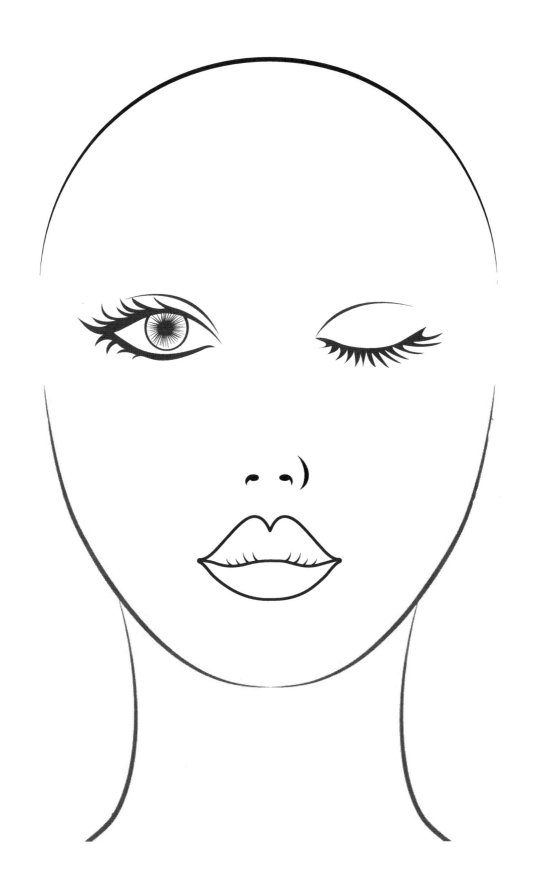

Skin preparation

Cleaning: ....

Scrubbing: ....

Lotion: ....

Moisturizing: ....

Base: ....

Foundation: ....

Correction: ....

Blush: ....

Powder: ....

Comments and advice

The eyes

Eyebrows: ....

Eyelids: ....

Pencil: ....

Mascara: ....

Liner: ....

The lips

Hydration: ....

balm ....

Gloss: ....

Pencil: ....

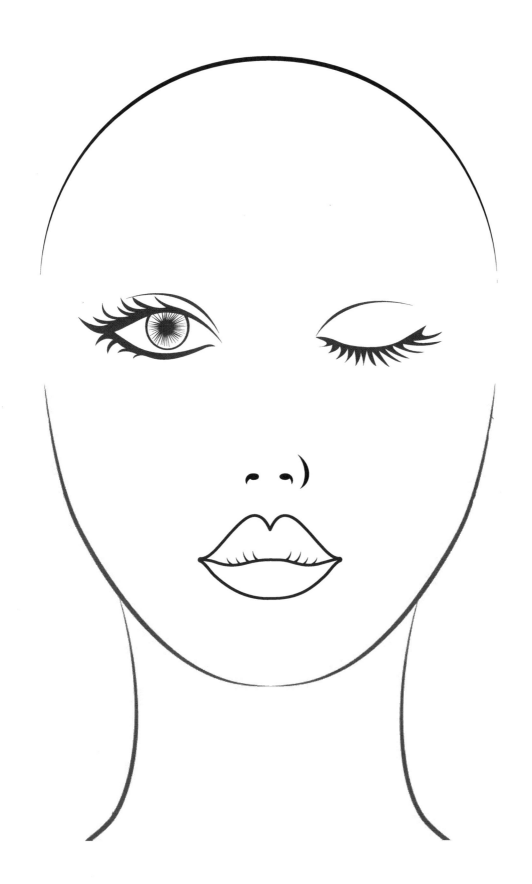

Skin preparation

Cleaning: ....

Scrubbing: ....

Lotion: ....

Moisturizing: ....

Base: ....

Foundation: ....

Correction: ....

Blush: ....

Powder: ....

Comments and advice

The eyes

Eyebrows: ....

Eyelids: ....

Pencil: ....

Mascara: ....

Liner: ....

The lips

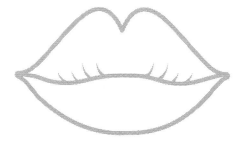

Hydration: ....

balm ....

Gloss: ....

Pencil: ....

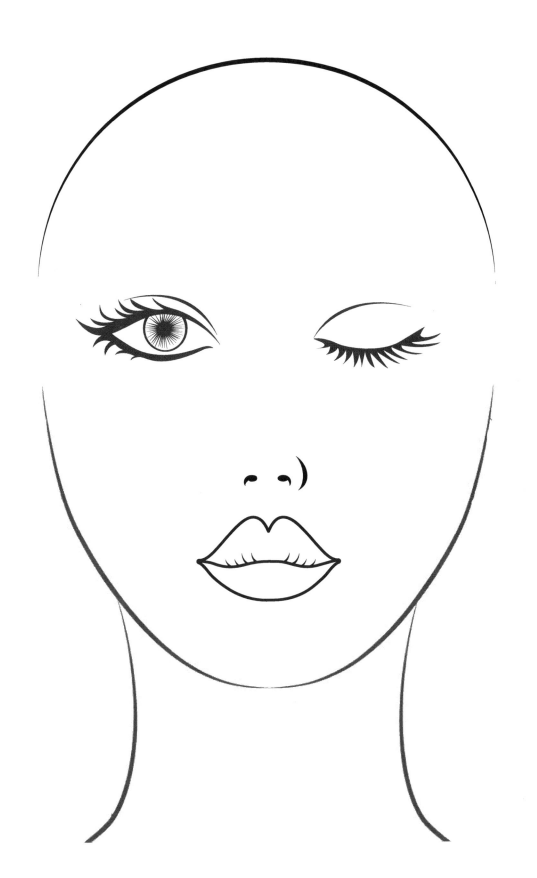

Skin preparation

Cleaning : _____

Scrubbing: _____

Lotion: _____

Moisturizing: _____

Base : _____

Foundation: _____

Correction: _____

Blush: _____

Powder: _____

Comments and advice

The eyes

Eyebrows: _____

Eyelids: _____

Pencil: _____

Mascara: _____

Liner : _____

The lips

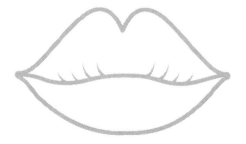

Hydration: _____

balm _____

Gloss: _____

Pencil: _____

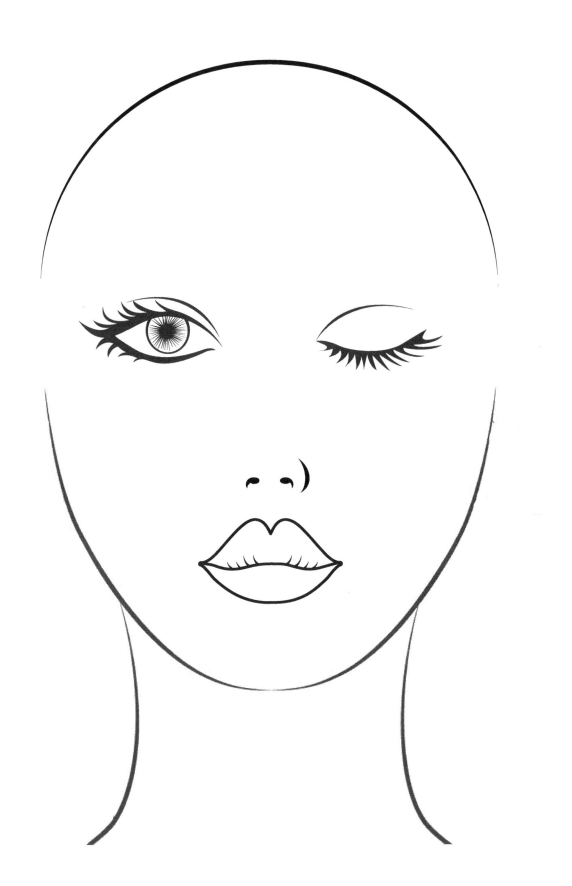

Skin preparation

Cleaning : ....

Scrubbing: ....

Lotion: ....

Moisturizing: ....

Base : ....

Foundation: ....

Correction: ....

Blush: ....

Powder: ....

Comments and advice

The eyes

Eyebrows: ....

Eyelids: ....

Pencil: ....

Mascara: ....

Liner : ....

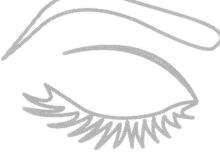

The lips

Hydration: ....

balm ....

Gloss: ....

Pencil: ....

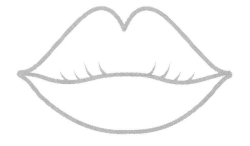

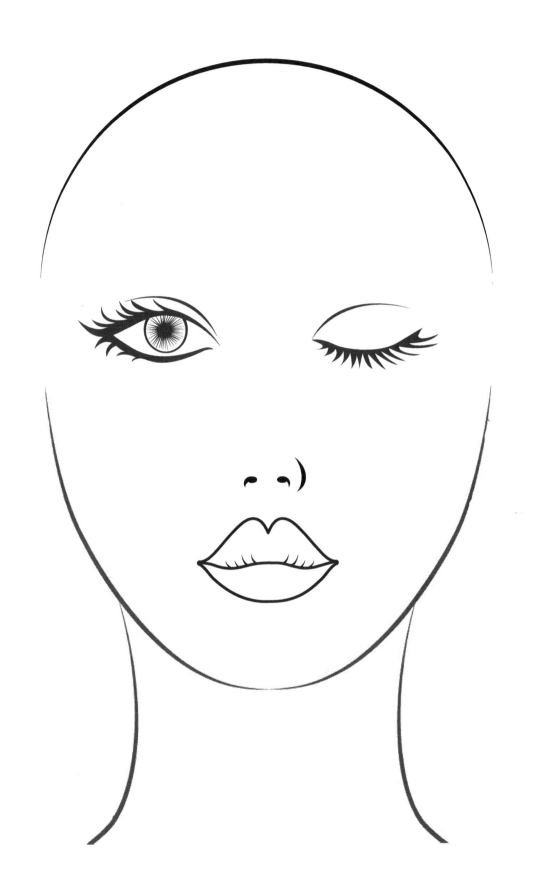

Skin preparation

Cleaning: _____

Scrubbing: _____

Lotion: _____

Moisturizing: _____

Base: _____

Foundation: _____

Correction: _____

Blush: _____

Powder: _____

Comments and advice

The eyes

Eyebrows: _____

Eyelids: _____

Pencil: _____

Mascara: _____

Liner: _____

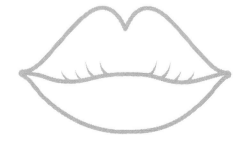

The lips

Hydration: _____

balm _____

Gloss: _____

Pencil: _____

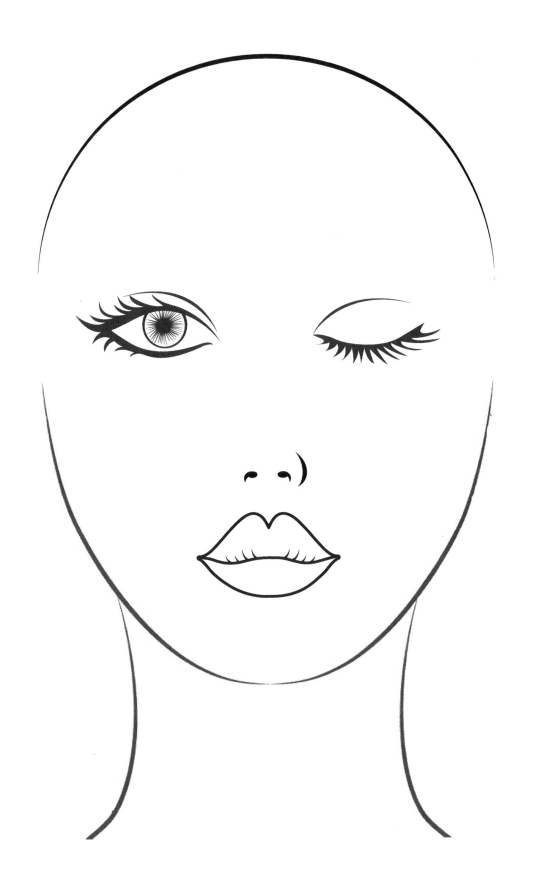

Skin preparation

Cleaning : _____
Scrubbing: _____
Lotion: _____
Moisturizing: _____
Base : _____
Foundation: _____
Correction: _____
Blush: _____
Powder: _____

Comments and advice

The eyes

Eyebrows: _____
Eyelids: _____
Pencil: _____
Mascara: _____
Liner : _____

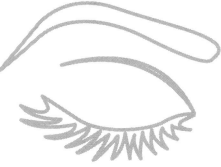

The lips

Hydration: _____
balm _____
Gloss: _____
Pencil: _____

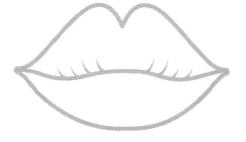

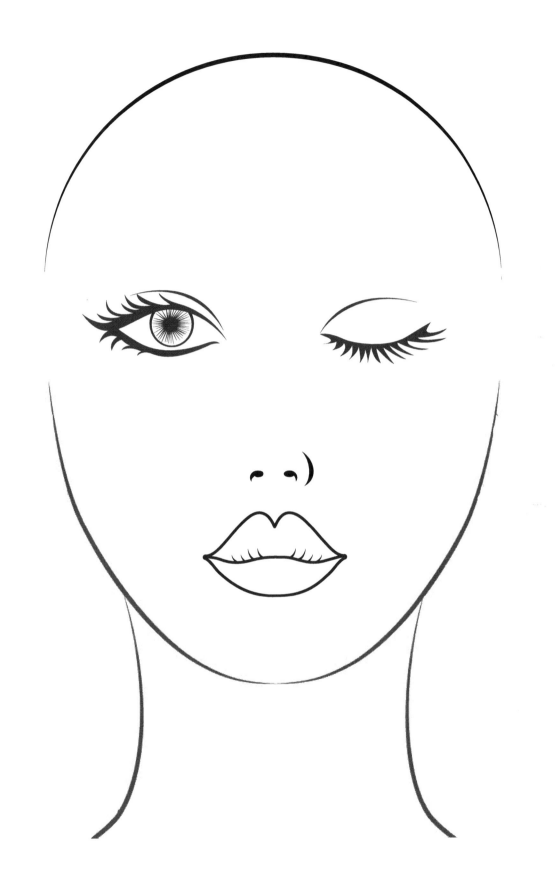

Skin preparation

Cleaning : _____
Scrubbing: _____
Lotion: _____
Moisturizing: _____
Base : _____
Foundation: _____
Correction: _____
Blush: _____
Powder: _____

Comments and advice

The eyes

Eyebrows: _____
Eyelids: _____
Pencil: _____
Mascara: _____
Liner : _____

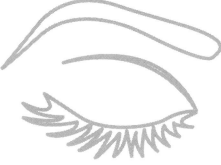

The lips

Hydration: _____
balm _____
Gloss: _____
Pencil: _____

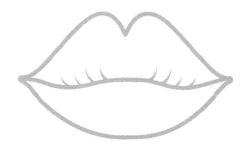

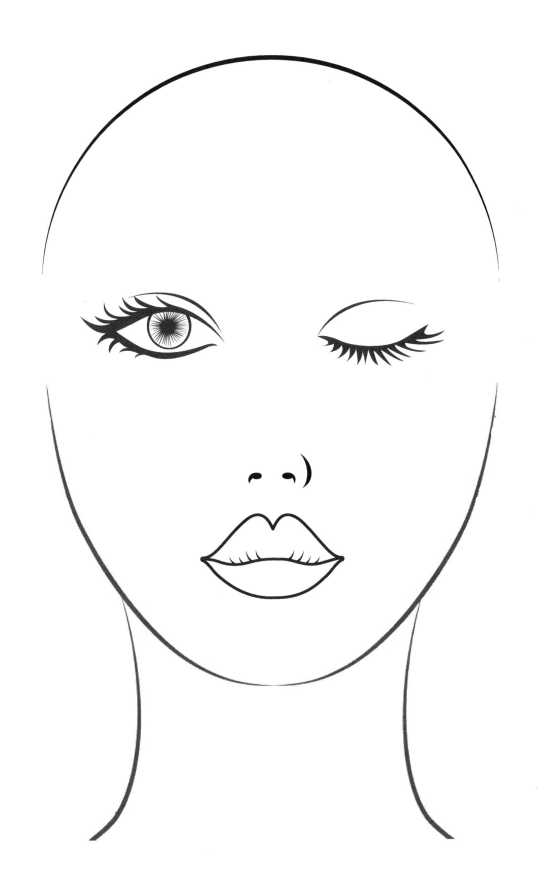

Skin preparation

Cleaning : _____
Scrubbing: _____
Lotion: _____
Moisturizing: _____
Base : _____
Foundation: _____
Correction: _____
Blush: _____
Powder: _____

Comments and advice

The eyes

Eyebrows: _____
Eyelids: _____
Pencil: _____
Mascara: _____
Liner : _____

The lips

Hydration: _____
balm _____
Gloss: _____
Pencil: _____

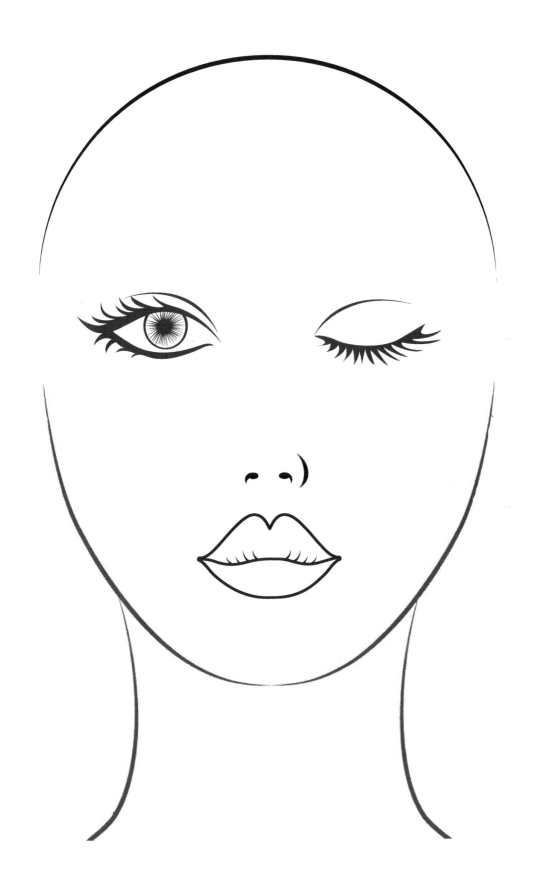

Skin preparation

Cleaning: ....

Scrubbing: ....

Lotion: ....

Moisturizing: ....

Base: ....

Foundation: ....

Correction: ....

Blush: ....

Powder: ....

Comments and advice

The eyes

Eyebrows: ....

Eyelids: ....

Pencil: ....

Mascara: ....

Liner: ....

The lips

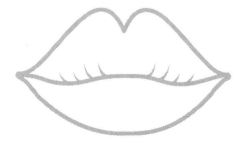

Hydration: ....

balm ....

Gloss: ....

Pencil: ....

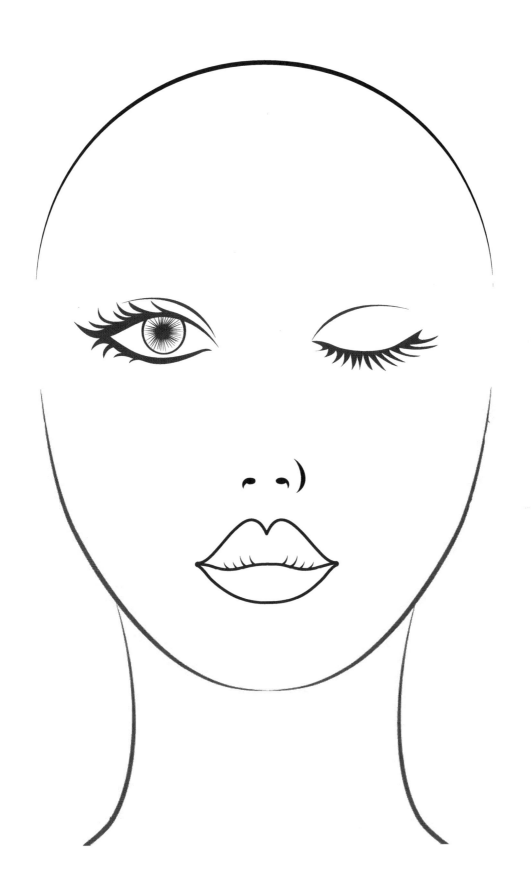

Skin preparation

Cleaning : _____

Scrubbing: _____

Lotion: _____

Moisturizing: _____

Base : _____

Foundation: _____

Correction: _____

Blush: _____

Powder: _____

Comments and advice

The eyes

Eyebrows: _____

Eyelids: _____

Pencil: _____

Mascara: _____

Liner : _____

The lips

Hydration: _____

balm _____

Gloss: _____

Pencil: _____

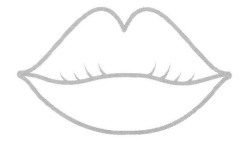

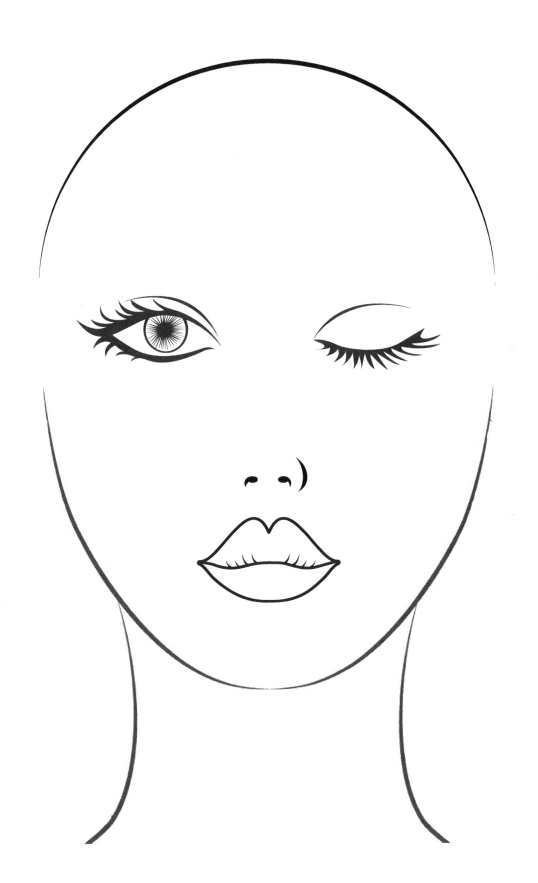

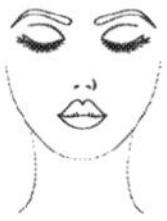

Skin preparation

Cleaning :

Scrubbing:

Lotion:

Moisturizing:

Base :

Foundation:

Correction:

Blush:

Powder:

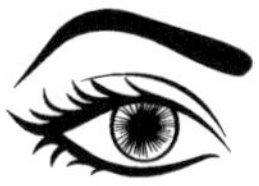

Comments and advice

The eyes

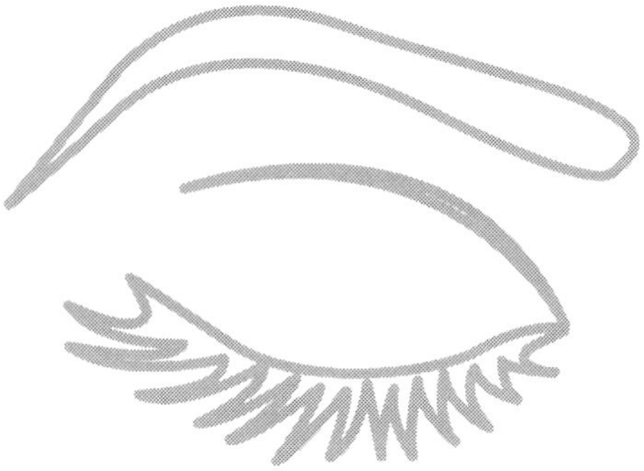

Eyebrows:

Eyelids:

Pencil:

Mascara:

Liner :

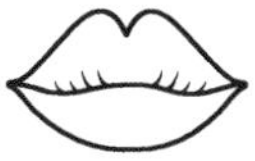

The lips

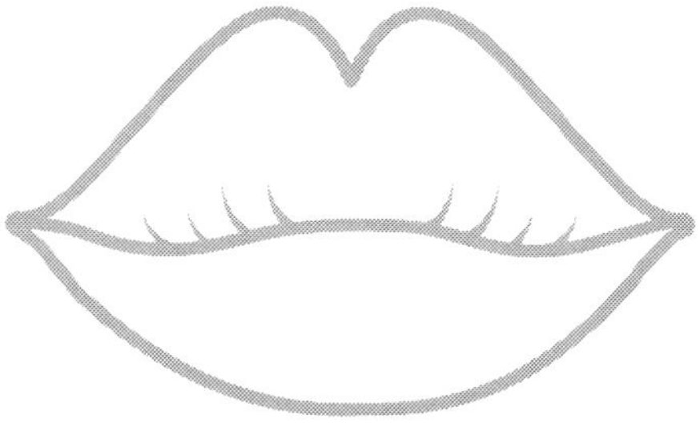

Hydration:

balm

Gloss:

Pencil:

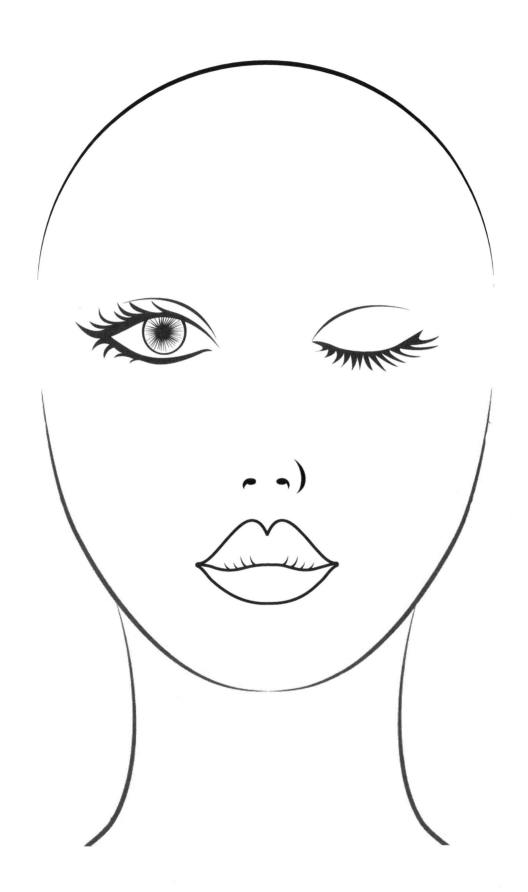

Skin preparation

Cleaning : ....

Scrubbing: ....

Lotion: ....

Moisturizing: ....

Base : ....

Foundation: ....

Correction: ....

Blush: ....

Powder: ....

Comments and advice

The eyes

Eyebrows: ....

Eyelids: ....

Pencil: ....

Mascara: ....

Liner : ....

The lips

Hydration: ....

balm ....

Gloss: ....

Pencil: ....

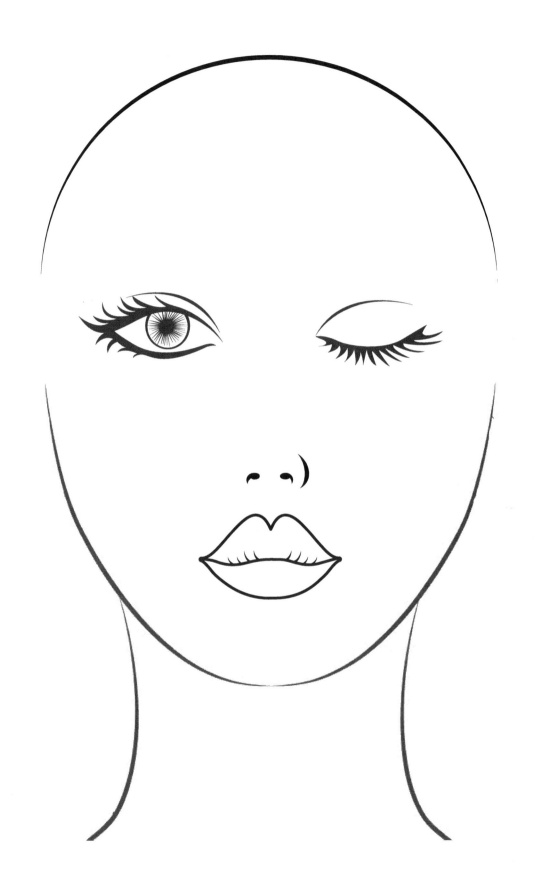

Skin preparation

Cleaning : _____
Scrubbing: _____
Lotion: _____
Moisturizing: _____
Base : _____
Foundation: _____
Correction: _____
Blush: _____
Powder: _____

Comments and advice

The eyes

Eyebrows: _____
Eyelids: _____
Pencil: _____
Mascara: _____
Liner : _____

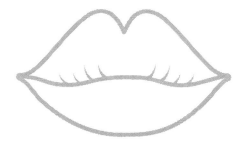

The lips

Hydration: _____
balm _____
Gloss: _____
Pencil: _____

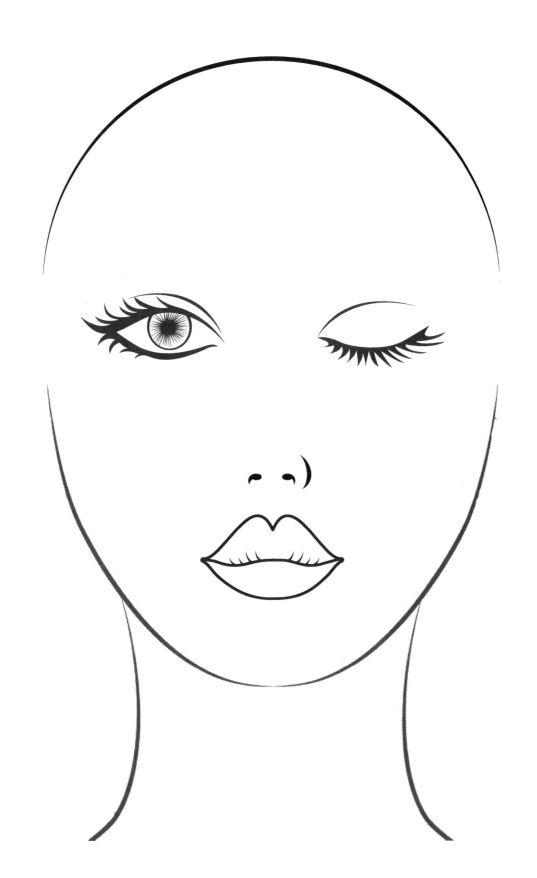

Skin preparation

Cleaning : ___
Scrubbing: ___
Lotion: ___
Moisturizing: ___
Base : ___
Foundation: ___
Correction: ___
Blush: ___
Powder: ___

Comments and advice

The eyes

Eyebrows: ___
Eyelids: ___
Pencil: ___
Mascara: ___
Liner : ___

The lips

Hydration: ___
balm ___
Gloss: ___
Pencil: ___

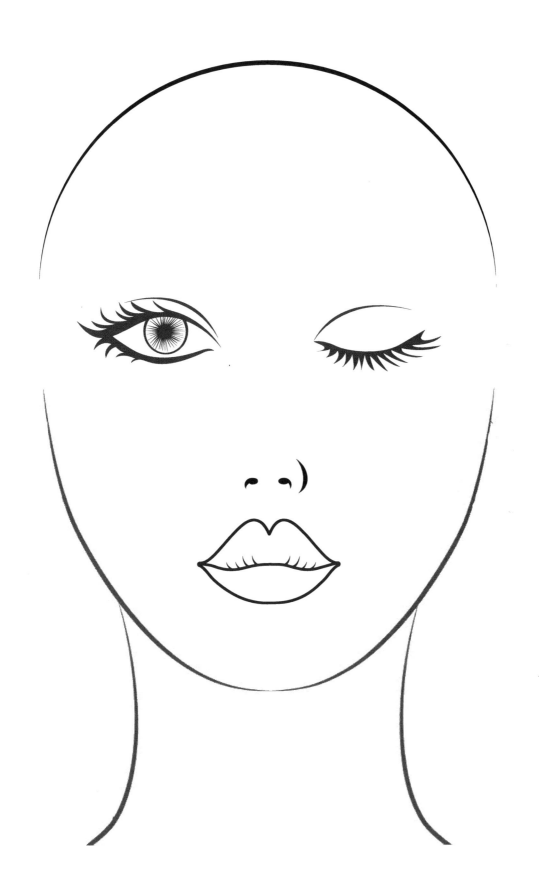

Skin preparation

Cleaning : _____
Scrubbing: _____
Lotion: _____
Moisturizing: _____
Base : _____
Foundation: _____
Correction: _____
Blush: _____
Powder: _____

Comments and advice

The eyes

Eyebrows: _____
Eyelids: _____
Pencil: _____
Mascara: _____
Liner : _____

The lips

Hydration: _____
balm _____
Gloss: _____
Pencil: _____

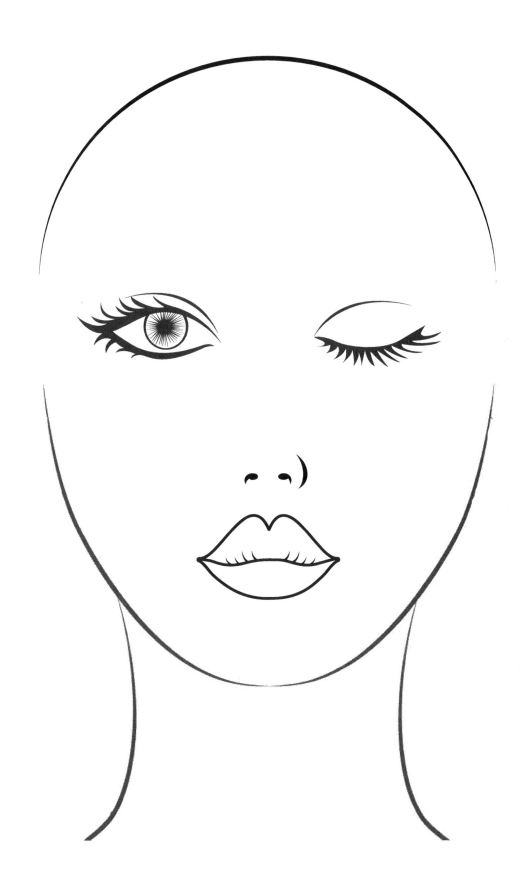

Skin preparation

Cleaning :
Scrubbing:
Lotion:
Moisturizing:
Base :
Foundation:
Correction:
Blush:
Powder:

Comments and advice

The eyes

Eyebrows:
Eyelids:
Pencil:
Mascara:
Liner :

The lips

Hydration:
balm
Gloss:
Pencil:

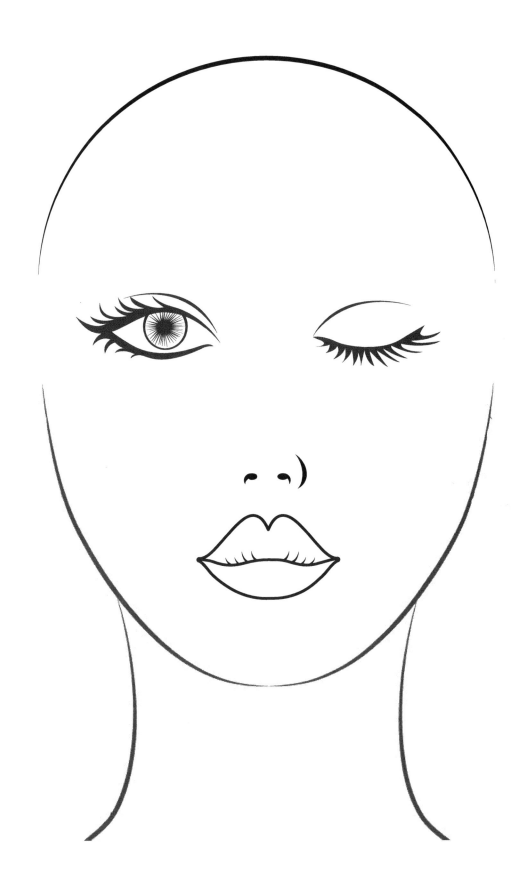

Skin preparation

Cleaning : _____

Scrubbing: _____

Lotion: _____

Moisturizing: _____

Base : _____

Foundation: _____

Correction: _____

Blush: _____

Powder: _____

Comments and advice

The eyes

Eyebrows: _____

Eyelids: _____

Pencil: _____

Mascara: _____

Liner : _____

The lips

Hydration: _____

balm _____

Gloss: _____

Pencil: _____

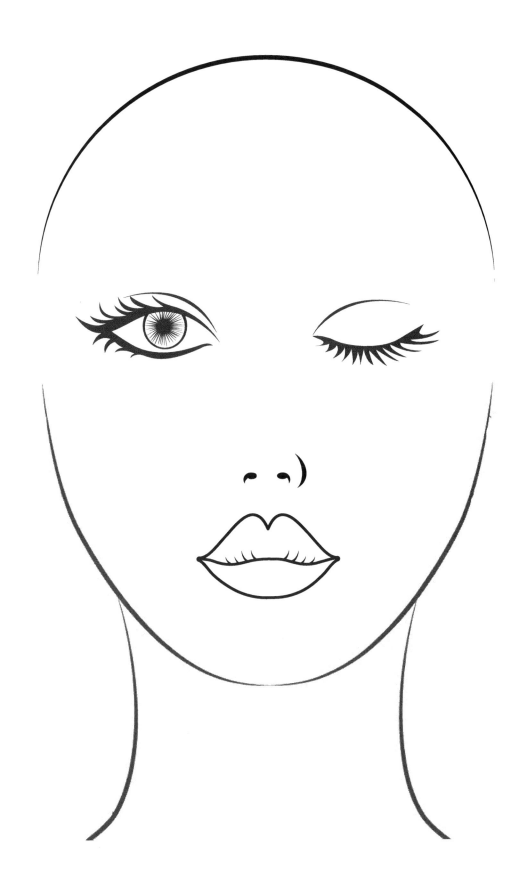

Skin preparation

Cleaning : _____
Scrubbing: _____
Lotion: _____
Moisturizing: _____
Base : _____
Foundation: _____
Correction: _____
Blush: _____
Powder: _____

Comments and advice

The eyes

Eyebrows: _____
Eyelids: _____
Pencil: _____
Mascara: _____
Liner : _____

The lips

Hydration: _____
balm _____
Gloss: _____
Pencil: _____

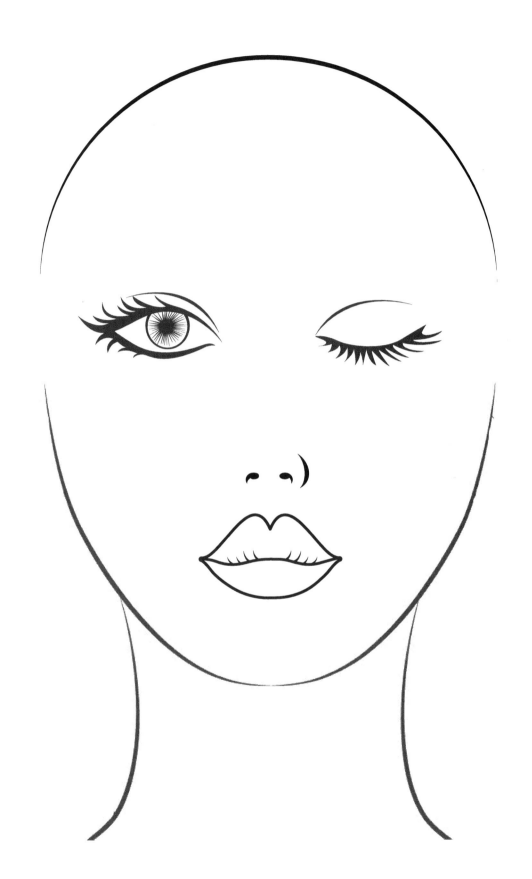

Skin preparation

Cleaning : ___
Scrubbing: ___
Lotion: ___
Moisturizing: ___
Base : ___
Foundation: ___
Correction: ___
Blush: ___
Powder: ___

Comments and advice

The eyes

Eyebrows: ___
Eyelids: ___
Pencil: ___
Mascara: ___
Liner : ___

The lips

Hydration: ___
balm ___
Gloss: ___
Pencil: ___

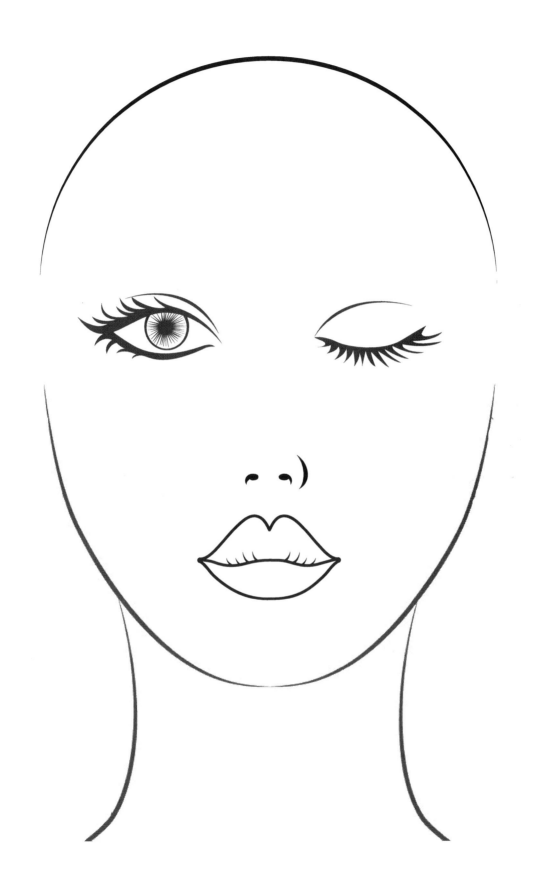

Printed in Great Britain
by Amazon

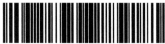